Call Sign:
DUSTOFF 34

Hovering Between Life and Death

Douglas (Doug) N Petersen (aka DUSTOFF 34)

Call Sign: DUSTOFF 34, Hovering Between Life and Death, by Douglas N Petersen. ISBN 978-1-63868-215-8 (softcover); 978-1-63868-216-5 (electronic).

Library of Congress Control Number: on file with Publisher.

Printed in the United States of America.

CONTENTS

DEDICATION

I dedicate this book to all my Brothers and Sisters whose names are etched on a black granite wall in Washington, DC, The Vietnam Veterans Memorial, "The Wall." I tried my best to avoid having your name etched on this memorial, but my best was not good enough. You are the true heroes of the Vietnam War. God rest your souls.

INTRODUCTION

Like many others before me, we write about one of the most traumatic times, and yet most meaningful times in our lives. These times were captured in our memory of the many months while serving in the US Army in Vietnam. This will be my accounting of the months leading up to and including my time there. It's now fifty-five years later, the memory has faded, details are not as sharp as they were, but this is what I recall as the truth as I remember.

The photos are not the best quality in some cases. The pictures from Vietnam were probably taken with a cheap camera I bought at the Post Exchange (PX) on Long Binh, possibly a Kodak Instamatic, I think. Capturing good quality photos was not high on my list of priorities. I didn't have or even want an expensive 35mm camera. I apologize for the poor quality. Most photos are mine, a couple are from another pilot, and one or two are from postings on Facebook, and the photographer is unknown to me. I'm just being up front about this.

Each chapter is dedicated to a specific time, a place or an event. As such, the chapter may be rather short and to the point. My intention is not to embellish with non-factual bullshit. I want it to be a succinct account of this period in my life. I have labeled some sections with "MISSION", as it will describe a very specific mission I flew. I flew hundreds of missions, not just the handful I write about in this book. Periodically, a thought will come to mind, and I will interject it into a section of the book. While it may not directly relate to the chapter, I wanted to include it. I mark these as "(Side Note)."

Let me define DUSTOFF. It is the call sign for the unarmed medical evacuation helicopter. We had a crew of four: aircraft commander (aka PIC, pilot-in-command), copilot (aka Peter Pilot), medic and crew chief. We were flying a UH-1H, Huey helicopter which was a single engine, two-bladed aircraft made by Bell Helicopter for the US Army. We had red crosses painted on a white background on each of the cargo doors, the nose of the helicopter and the bottom. It was clearly marked as to what our mission was.

The Huey 'schoolbook solution' for the configuration for a medical evacuation mission was for two jump seats for the medic and crew chief and hanging straps for 3 litters. Well, that's all fine and dandy in a controlled environment, but in a combat zone, being shot at, we didn't have the time to follow that configuration. I seldom used the 3 litters, because of the time it took to load a patient and trying the get the upper litter in the hooks that were over the head of the crew chief and medic was extremely difficult. Can you imagine lifting 250 pounds above your head while knee deep in rice paddy water? Also, in the school book solution, the jump seats only took up too much space, so these were removed. The crew in the back usually sat on a cushion and we would load as many causalities as we could fit in the space. ARVN's (Army of the Republic of Vietnam) were usually small individuals, and we could carry quite a few on each mission. The record for me on a mission was 34, including the crew. We were very heavy that day. How did you do that, you may ask? On each side of the rotor transmission (called the 'hell-hole') there was a small bench seat, designed for two people. We had 9 in each hell-hole, 3 sitting down, 3 on their laps, and 3 more facing them and then we slid the cargo door shut. The rest of the injured were in the center cargo area.

I said that we were 'unarmed' meaning that the aircraft did not have any mounted weapons. Typically, the two pilots had a side arm, mine was a .38 caliber, Smith & Wesson revolver. The crew chief and medic had a side arm and probably a M-16 rifle. The point that I need to make is that while we had weapons, these were strictly for patient protection and not to be used in an offensive role, strictly defensive. Also remember, we didn't have time to engage the enemy. The medic and crew chief were busy taking care of the injured and didn't have time to engage the enemy. The pilots were busy too, getting the aircraft and crew away from the enemy fire.

Almost every DUSTOFF mission was flown as a single aircraft. We very seldom had any other aircraft with us as we flew our missions. We flew day and night, good weather or bad, it made no difference. We're out there in very remote places, all by ourselves, taking care of business.

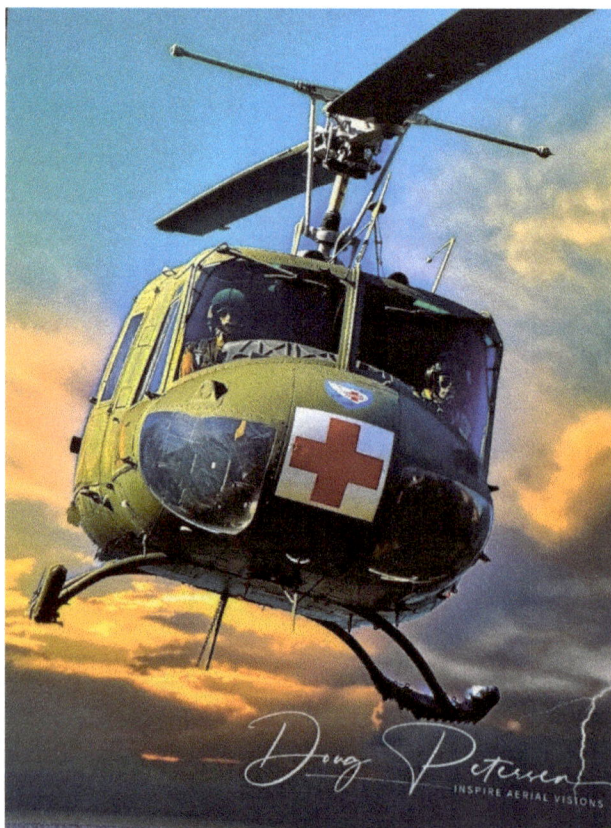

Most of the DUSTOFF missions I will describe, I probably won't remember any of the crew member's names. And none of the missions will I recall the names of the injured we picked up to take to a medical facility. I wish I did, but I don't. Remember, we're in a combat zone and asking for the injured soldier's name and Social Security Number wasn't an option. We needed to get the injured on board the helicopter, begin medical treatment, and get them to a medical facility, all the while being shot at many times.

Record keeping of individual flights by the crew was nonexistent and the records in the unit weren't very good either. Back then, to be honest, it wasn't important. I was a 22-year-old kid and did not think I would want the information 55 years later. How many missions did I fly? I have no idea. What I do know is that I am credited with nearly 1,000 combat flight hours for my tour. It is also estimated that each crew in a normal tour in Vietnam would have evacuated almost 1,300 patients.

In the upcoming pages, I will describe specific missions that stand out in my memory. While there are only six written in detail, I flew hundreds of missions during my tour, just like every other Dustoff crew who flew this mission. Some descriptions are short, remember I promised I will not embellish with nonfactual bullshit just to put words on paper or words in a book.

The missions will be titled with the approximate grid map coordinates of the mission. Some of these

5

PZ's are still marked with grease pencil on my map I have. These will not make any sense to most of you, and it's not to confuse or distract from my description of the mission. It is merely to give context to what we were experiencing. We did not use latitude and longitude for coordinates of our pickup zones; we had grid markings on our maps (you can see that from my map on an upcoming page). Also keep in mind, we relied on our map, and our visual navigation skills to find these locations. We didn't use navigation radios and certainly did not have GPS.

One point I mention later in the book and on the TEDx San Antonio talk I gave, is that there are no weekends in war. There aren't holidays where we don't have missions to fly. We flew seven days a week, twenty-four hours a day, in good weather or bad. We were there to get the injured to a place where they could receive treatment. Imagine if we had a "CLOSED Sunday" sign on the door.

Before I go any further, I believe you, the reader needs to know some basic information about DUSTOFF.

- During the almost 11-year Vietnam War (1962 – 1973), American helicopter crews, known as Dustoff, evacuated some 900,000 people to safety. This is more than the population of major cities in the United States.
- Of the nearly 496,000 combat missions flown, many were flown at night. We

flew in all weather conditions. Neither deterred us from flying the mission.

- Our aircrew loss was 33%. For me, this means that 1 out of 3 missions I flew I could be killed or wounded.

- Of the approximately 1,400 Dustoff pilots during the eleven years, 90 were killed and 380 were wounded and the lost ratio of the approximately 2,000 Dustoff medics and crew chiefs was 33%.

- The likelihood we would take enemy fire on any particular mission was probably greater than 50%, though I don't have a specific source for that number.

- During this timeframe, approximately 8,000 hoist missions were conducted. These were seven times more dangerous than any other mission. (More will be discussed in the book.)

- "The Golden Hour" refers to the time from injury to a medical facility and 98% of the "URGENT" missions arrived within that hour, significantly increasing their survival.

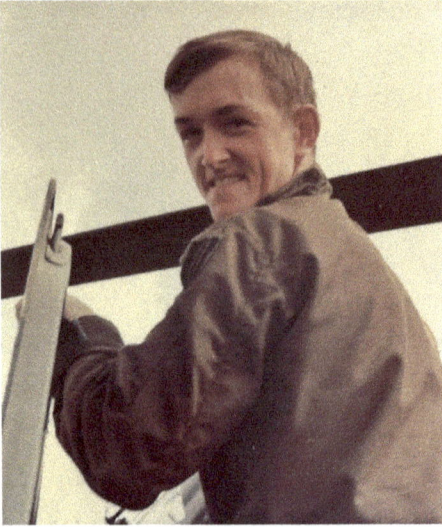

Lastly, I am not a hero. I was a young man, 22 years old, who wanted to serve our country as best I could, and I did it by flying as a DUST-OFF pilot.

VMI

It was the fall 1967 and I was beginning my college career at Virginia Military Institute, VMI. I'm not sure why I wanted so badly to go to VMI, but I did and after two attempts to get in, I was finally accepted. None of my family went there so it could have been any number of reasons I was so determined to attend this college.

My life at VMI is not the purpose of this book, but it lays the groundwork for the beginning of my interest in flying helicopters. I liked the military lifestyle of VMI, the discipline, the regiment, and the comraderies of fellow classmates, Brother Rats. I was sure I was on a military path of some sort.

We seldom got to watch television and keep up with the news. We were too busy with academics, parade practice, working off demerits (yes, I got some of those too), and whatever else that kept cadets busy. At some point I did get to see a little of what was going on and I'm certain while watching the news, it was about the war in Vietnam and a huge enemy campaign called the Tet of '68. Much has been written about Tet, but since I wasn't there, I can't go into much detail about it.

It was during this time I was beginning to see the role of the helicopter in Vietnam, and it sparked an interest, which grew into an obsession. I wanted to fly helicopters. After finishing three semesters and a summer school session, I had made the decision to leave VMI in the winter of 1969 to join the US Army. The Army at that time had a "high school to flight school" program. How I came to know this is a mystery, but I did. If I could pass a flight physical and a flight aptitude test, I could enlist into the Warrant Officer Candidate Flight School Program.

Much to the disappointment of my parents, I left VMI, came home and began preparing to join the US Army to fly helicopters. I was fully aware this decision would eventually lead me to Vietnam, and I was okay with that. My obsession to fly helicopters outweighed that concern. April 29, 1969, I raised my right hand and took an oath to serve our country, thus it began.

BASIC TRAINING & FLIGHT SCHOOL

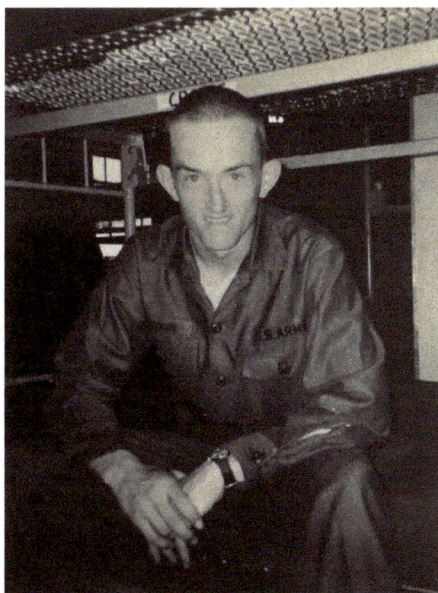

I don't remember how I left Richmond, VA, after I was sworn in, it must have been by bus to Fort Polk, Louisiana where I began my basic training. It was early May 1969 and already hot and muggy in Louisiana. My basic training company was Alpha Company, 1st Battalion, 1st Brigade, A-1-1 and a good number of us in that company were going to be Warrant Officer Candidates (WOC) after basic training in flight school.

11

During the 6- or 8-week training, our company was assigned the duty to provide a funeral service detail. To be selected, we went through some internal drill and ceremony competition. With my background from Hargrave Military Academy (I didn't talk about this previously) and VMI, I was selected. During my time at basic training, I did 2 or 3 funeral details in the local area. And darn, I missed pugil stick training.

Graduation from basic training at Fort Polk, LA, behind me now, it was time to move onto the next

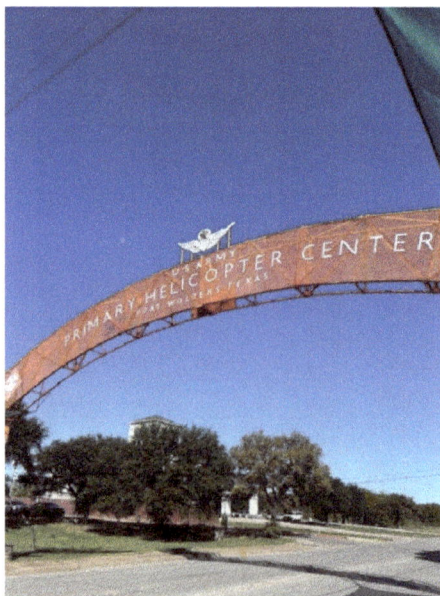

stage of my military career. I got on a bus and headed west to Texas. The bus pulled into Mineral Wells, Texas and exited Highway 180 to drive under the arch, "U.S. Army Primary Helicopter Training Center", Fort Wolters, Texas. It was the first week of July 1969. We pulled up to the barracks and were met by our new cadre. I was in the 5th Warrant Officer Candidate (WOC) Company, 70-5. (Though Fort Wolters no longer exits, the arch and two training helicopters are still there.)

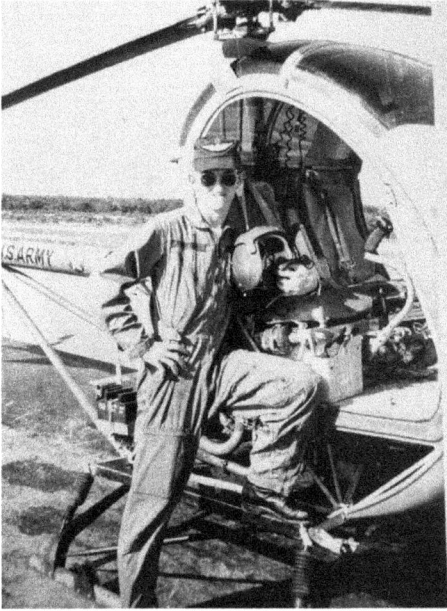

The training helicopter that I flew was the TH-55A, a very small two-seat aircraft. My instructor was "Pink Slip" Sergeant. He was known to hand out "pink slips" for unsatisfactory training flights frequently, and I am sure I got one or two.

I soloed pretty much on track with the others, not first and not last. After you soloed, the bus on the way back to the barracks would stop at the Holiday Inn and you would be thrown into the swimming pool. Also, the local car dealership would be happy to sell you a car. The reason you had to solo first was they had to be certain you were going to make it through the training. So off I go to Ed Lee Chevrolet in Mineral Wells and bought a used Ford Cortina (an English car… not very reliable, but it was all I could afford and I'm sure they wanted to get rid of it.)

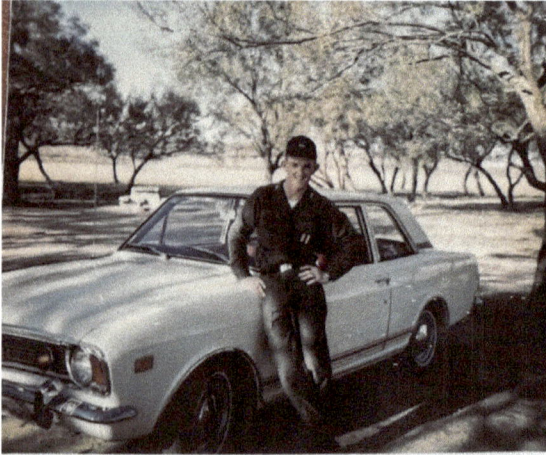

The red racing stripe on the door panel was included; it made it look like it was going faster than it really was.

The last picture of this section is our class photo at Fort Wolters before leaving for Fort Rucker, AL. Little did any of us know, two classmates in that photo would not come home as most of us did and be killed in action in the next twelve months. WO1 Frank Crouse would be killed flying a low observation helicopter in July 1970, engaging the enemy. The helicopter crashed and burned, killing him and the other pilot. WO1 Paul Brass was killed December 1970, flying a Dustoff mission, at night, in bad weather to pick up an injured soldier. They crashed into the side of a mountain, killing the entire crew. RIP my Brothers.

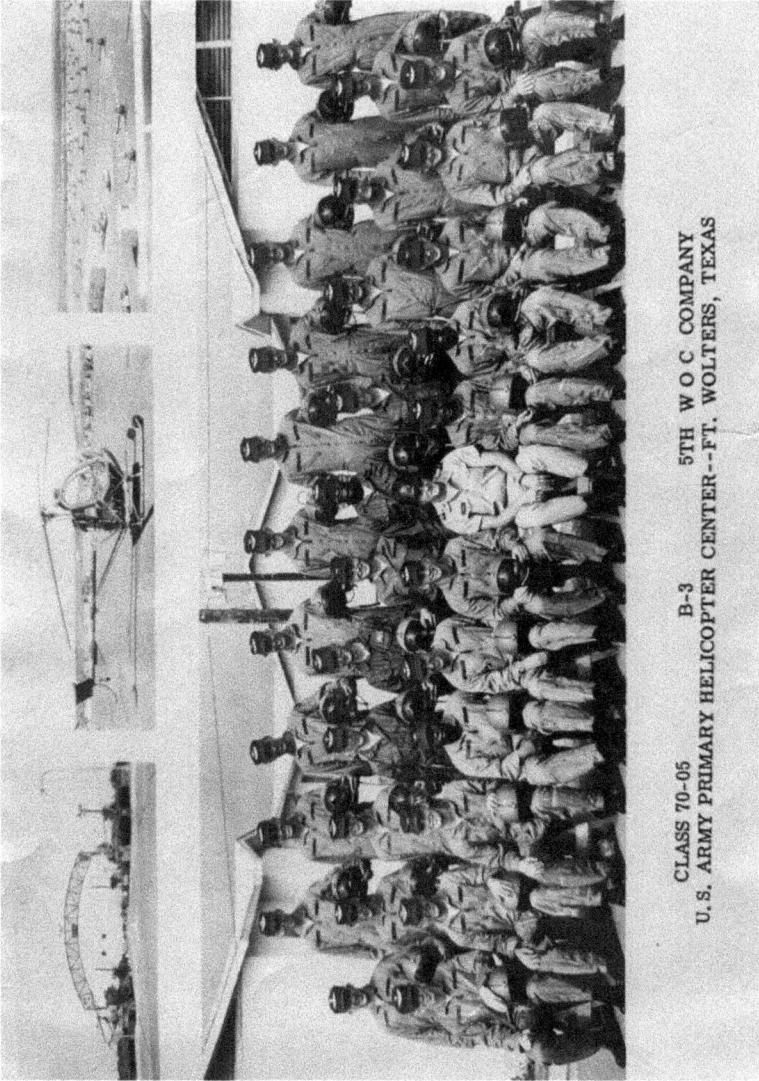

CLASS 70-05 B-3 5TH W O C COMPANY
U.S. ARMY PRIMARY HELICOPTER CENTER--FT. WOLTERS, TEXAS

15

Graduation from Fort Wolters was in early December and since the Army schools would be shut down during the upcoming holidays, I went back home

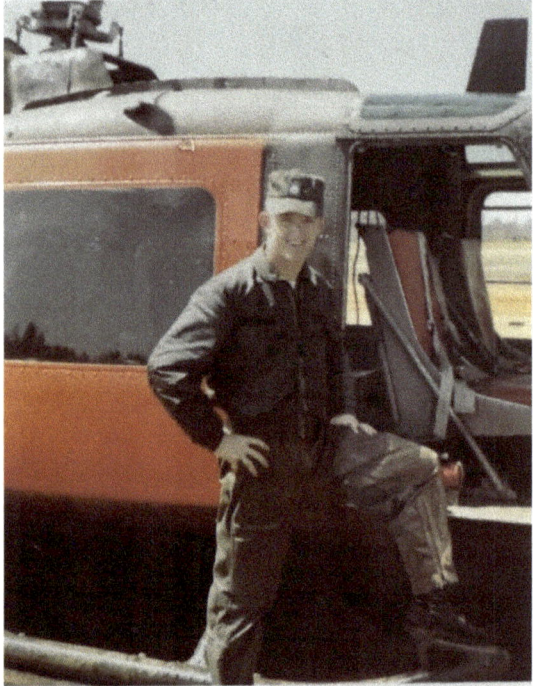

to Virginia Beach in my little Ford Cortina until the beginning of January 1970 to continue my training at Fort Rucker, Alabama. This is where we would begin flying the UH-1, Huey.

We did all sorts of advanced training now, learning to fly by instruments in the simulator and in the OH-13, and then began to fly the UH-1.

Beginning in April 1970, several of my classmates and I were selected to train in UH-1B gunships. The armament configurations were different from one helicopter to another, but we flew them all: twin mini-guns firing between 2,500 – 4,000 rounds per minute, or twin 2.75-inch rockets, or the 40mm grenade launcher. It was a blast shooting up all sorts of trucks and such down range. I was now a gun pilot.

Early May 1970, I was promoted from Warrant Officer Candidate (WOC) to Warrant Officer 1 (WO-1) and the next day awarded my U.S. Army Aviator badge. Almost one year to the date from swearing into the military to graduating from flight school. My smile was a mile wide.

OFF TO WAR

My memory of going over to Vietnam is rather vague. We had a layover at Fort Ord, California for a day, or an hour, I can't say for certain. We boarded a contract airline, probably Flying Tiger Airlines and off to Guam to refuel. I'm pretty sure it was a short layover there. Then we landed at Tan Son Nhut Air Force Base just outside of Saigon.

Without question, and many others will say the same thing, as we walked off the aircraft, down the boarding stairs, the first thing that hits you is the heat, and then the smell. The heat you can imagine, but the smell is hard to describe, much less than anything you could imagine. It wasn't pleasant.

Next stop was the 90th Replacement Battalion in Long Binh, Vietnam. This is where we would have a few days for indoctrination, start our malaria pill regiment, and wait for our assignments.

It was at the 90th where we converted our US currency to MPC (Military Payment Certificates). We wouldn't be using "greenback" money while in Vietnam.

While at the 90th, we were in direct flight path of a medical evacuation helicopter unit, and we could see them fly overhead to a hospital just over the barbed-wire fence. It was now getting real, very quickly. I was in a war zone.

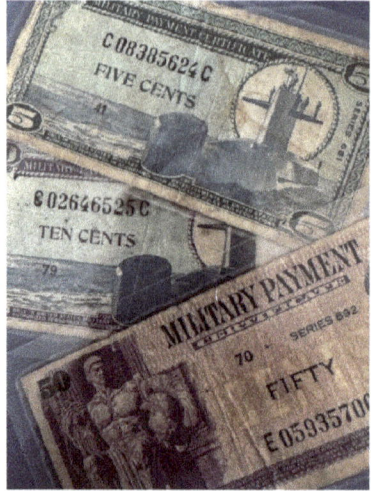

Now it was my turn to get my assignment, and a staff member told me I was being assigned to the 45th Medical Company (Air Ambulance) as a DUSTOFF pilot. I spoke up immediately and said, "You don't understand, I am a gunship guy." And the staff member looked at me and said, "No. You're a DUSTOFF guy now."

Shocked that all that gunship training I did in flight school was now to be characterized as just being a fun few weeks. It was now getting real. And wouldn't you know it, the 45th Med Co. was the helicopter unit that had been flying overhead, so my drive to my unit was quite short. In fact, I could have walked if it hadn't been for all the barbed wire.

(Side Note) This is a good point to mention that when I was sent over to Vietnam, I was on a general assignment order, and not to a specific unit. Many of the young pilots graduating from Fort Rucker, AL who were being assigned to a Dustoff unit were sent TDY (temporary duty) to Fort Sam Houston, TX to attend the US Army Medical Department (AMEDS) training program. This was a 6-week course covering all sorts of medical training from inoculations, learning to suture, open airways with a cricothyroidotomy, clean and debride wounds and more. But I didn't go to Fort Sam, remember, I didn't need this training, I was a "gunship guy."

45ᵀᴴ MEDICAL COMPANY (AIR AMBULANCE)

The 45th Medical Company was one of two full size medical helicopter companies in Vietnam. It was deployed from

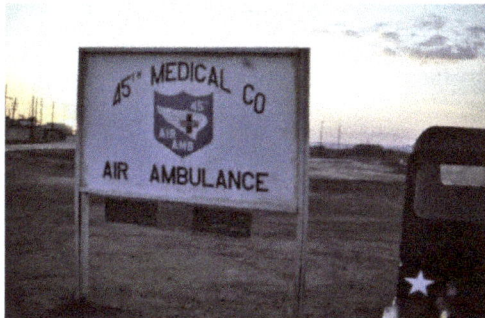

Photo credit: Unknown from Facebook

Fort Bragg, NC and became fully operational September 13, 1967, in Long Binh, Vietnam. A company size unit had 25 UH-1H "Huey" helicopters, and 4 platoons of pilots, medics, crew chiefs, admin staff, maintenance personnel, and the company dog (yes there was a dog in the company area but wasn't on the books as best I know.)

With all my gear in hand, I checked in to company headquarters and was led to my new home for the next 11 months. We called our living/sleeping space a 'hooch'. It was a room about 15 feet by 15 feet, and a small room in the back with a set of bunk beds. It did not have air conditioning when I walked through the door, and with the heat and humidity, it was critical to get one.

My first roommate was a Texan from Amarillo. His name was Jerry Ham. He and I began the process taking an empty shell of a hooch into something that was livable. We built a small bar in the living space and of course had our posters of Raquel Welch and another Playmate on the wall. At some point Jerry moved to another hooch with some other pilots and then would eventually take another assignment with another DUSTOFF unit. Sadly, Jerry died in 2009 in his hometown of Amarillo, Texas from a heart attack. RIP roomie.

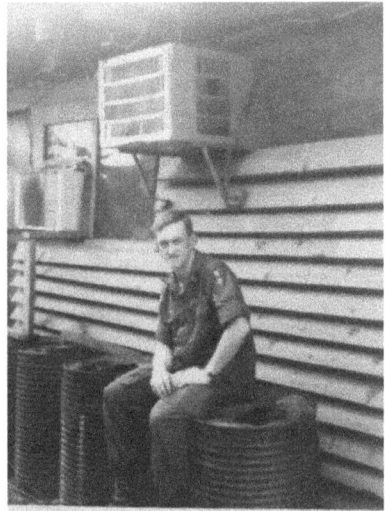

We needed an air conditioner and since there wasn't a Lowe's or Home Depot within walking distance, (that's a joke) we had to find someone who had an extra one and trade them for something we had and they wanted and in return, we would get an A/C unit. I don't remember what we traded, but we had cool air finally.

Speaking of trading… money was not used that much. If you wanted something, then you would most likely have to trade someone for it. For instance, I wanted a pair of Australian kangaroo boots, I don't remember who had them or what I traded, but I got them. Let me say, I wore those boots for many years, the best boots I ever wore. I was given 4 or 5 map sheets of our area of operation. Once I taped them together, marked the grid lines and numbers, it needed to be covered with lamination. So, I found a source and found something to trade. Now I had my map. We needed the maps to be laminated because we would write mission data with a grease pencil and would wipe them off when completed. If you look closely at the picture of the map below, you can still see some of the markings I made for missions I flew.

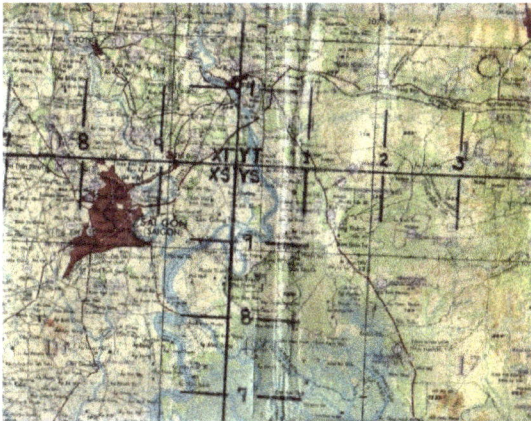

During the first few days with the 45th, I would fly with a senior pilot for an orientation of the area, check my pilot proficiency, and then put into the flight schedule. I believe my first flight I took was with another Warrant Officer, Bob Bixby. He was one of the instructor pilots in the unit.

LONG BINH

As I previously mentioned, the 45th Med Co was based out of Long Binh. We had three crews on standby 24 hours a day, 7 days a week. These crews were responsible to fly missions in a designated area around the home base. "First Up" crew would be launched for first mission that was called in the area around Long Binh. Typically, we would be restricted to our company area until the alert horn would sound and then we would rush to the helicopter. The sequence as I recall was, the crew chief would untie the rotor blade and get ready for engine start. The copilot would jump in the right seat and start the engine. The medic would be assisting as needed. The AC, aircraft commander, aka. Pilot-In-Command (PIC) would get the mission, run to the helicopter on the "First Up" helicopter pad, put on a chest chicken plate, and survival vest and then climb into the left seat and strap in. After seated, the AC would assume the aircraft controls while the copilot finished getting his chicken plate and survival vest

27

on and strapped into his seat. This took place in two minutes.

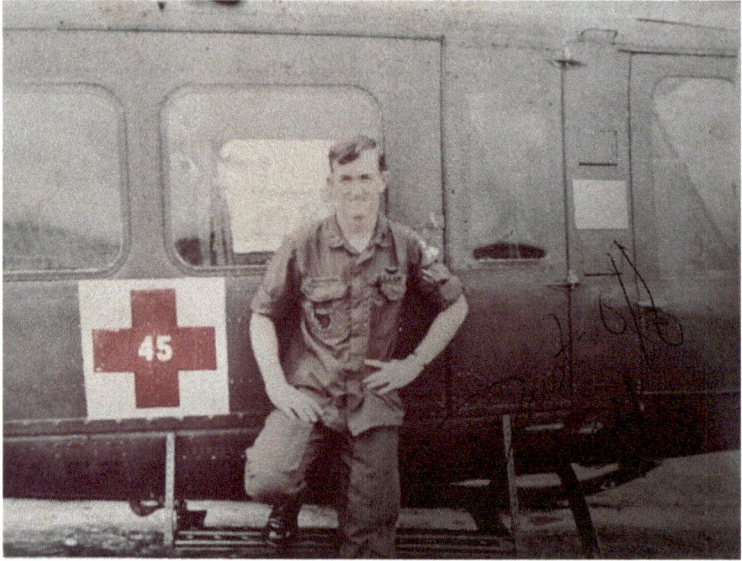

"Second Up" was another crew who was ready to take the next mission if "First Up" was out on their mission. The same time constraints applied to this crew. "Third Up" was an admin crew. This crew would transfer medical equipment or pick up blood from one hospital to another. Occasionally, this crew would be launched for a mission if the other two crews were out.

(Side Note) Pilots have this unique ability to compartmentalize their environment and situation. We can prioritize what is going on around us and put them into compartments so as not to interfere with the highest priority. One example I recall was I was flying 3rd Up and flying a mission between Saigon and one of the hospitals at Long Binh and a radio call came over to the air for us. The RTO (Radio Telephone Operator) asked if I was on board. We acknowledged, 'Affirmative'. The RTO said to relay a message to him that his grandmother has passed away. Probably not the most sensitive decision to convey that message to me, but that's the way it happened. We continued the mission and when I had some down time, I would process it later. Remember, communicating with family in the states was limited to letters, or setting up a MARS (Military Affiliate Radio System) call. Both were not the most efficient communications.

(Side Note) Bob Hope, Ann Margaret, and other Hollywood celebrities were part of the USO tour, and they were doing their Christmas show in Long Binh in December 1970. I was 1st Up, so I wouldn't be attending the show. The area around the show was a designated 'no fly zone'. Well, the mission horn sounded, it was an "URGENT" mission, and we were off to evacuate another injured soldier. Looking at the coordinates of the pickup zone, our location, it was clear that I would violate the 'no fly zone' since the shortest distance between two points is a straight line. Admittingly, we violated the 'no fly zone' airspace. (Feel free to report me if you'd like. I mean, what would they do? Send me to Vietnam?) Later, as I watched a recording of the show, you can hear a helicopter passing by and Bob Hope making some sort of comment… yep, it was me. So, I can now say I was on the USO Bob Hope Show!

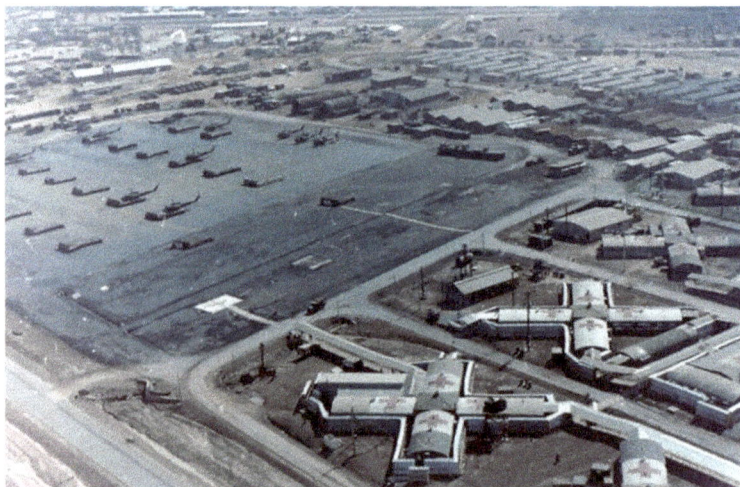

Long Binh has two major hospitals, 93rd Evacuation Hospital and the 24th Surgical Hospital. Depending on the patient's injury, it would dictate which hospital we would take them. As seen in the photo above, the 45th (on the upper left) was adjacent to the 93rd Evac (on the lower right). Some of the nurses who were assigned with the 93rd would come over to socialize with us from time to time. The nurses from the 24th seemed to be more interested in the doctors over there and not the pilots at the 45th.

Not all missions could be flown out of the home base in Long Binh because the flight time from there to the pickup zone would jeopardize the life of the wounded soldier. Our total area of operation was massive, so we also operated out of four remote sites. These remote sites the crew would spend four days at a time and fly that area of operation. We called these 'Standby'. Having a crew closer to the injured would help get them to a medical facility for treatment and meet the "Golden Hour." The remote sites were, Tay Ninh, Tan An, Nui Dat, and Xuan Loc. Each one was unique in their own way.

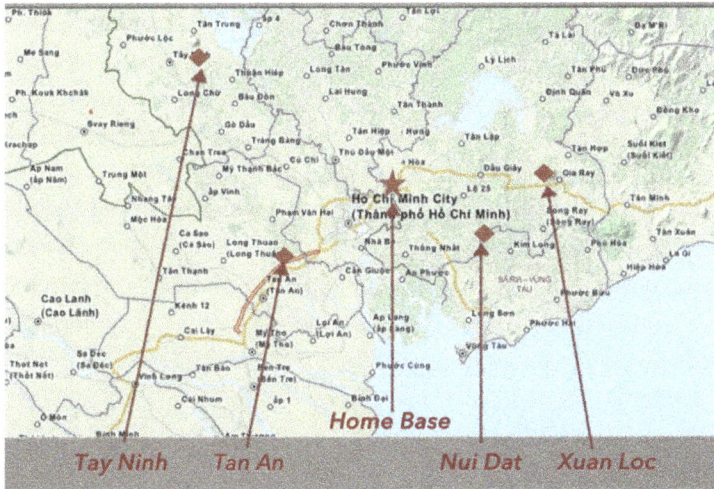

Before I get into more detail about each of these standby locations, it would be important to discuss the various types of pick-up zones.

The western half of our area of operation was relatively flat terrain. There were a lot of rice paddies and open fields. When we got into the vicinity of the pick-up zone, we could clearly see the best approach path and the best exit route. As previously mentioned, we would fly at an altitude minimizing small arms enemy fire, then do some crazy-ass maneuver to drop out of the sky quickly to get down to a low-level profile. Flying at 90-100 knots, about

5-10 feet above the ground we approached the pick-up zone, flared the helicopter to bring it to a halt to land. Flaring the helicopter too much the tail rotor might strike the ground, so you really needed to be mindful of the surroundings. Another maneuver that would help dissipate the airspeed was a side flare. Another tricky maneuver, but we learned.

We would touchdown as close to the patients we could. Maybe it was the rice paddy dyke, or even in the mud. Wherever it was, we would be on the ground for about two to three minutes loading the injured. We wanted to minimize time of the ground for two reasons, one to get the injured to a medical facility as quick as we could and second to reduce the time the enemy could shoot at us.

I'm not sure if I landed on a US Navy river boat on one of my missions, but I do know others that did. Whether I flew on one of those missions, I'm not sure.

The next pick-up zone type was a "hover down." These were generally in our eastern area of operation. The PZ was too small just to fly in and fly out because to the jungle conditions. It was big enough for our helicopter, but barely. As we would approach the top of the jungle, the crew chief, on one side and the medic on the other, would stick their heads out the cargo door to make sure the tail rotor was clear of obstacles. Slowly and methodically, I would descend, taking direction from the crew in the back on which way to turn my tail rotor to keep it clear from hitting a tree. All the while, I am watching the main rotor to make sure it doesn't turn into a weedwhacker with the jungle in front of us. Just a point of interest, the main rotor blades of a Huey are thin-skinned and do not like chopping trees. Once damaged, the flight back, even, if possible, would be rough.

On our "hover down" missions our exposure to the enemy was longer, usually 10 minutes or so and exiting would take almost as much time as it did in descending.

The last PZ I will discuss is where we couldn't land at all and required us to do a hoist mission. Here we would hover just above the jungle, lower a jungle penetrator down to the ground on a cable to load the injured. I will go into more detail in an upcoming chapter just on hoist missions. Our exposure time in a hoist mission was 20-30 minutes, just hovering over the jungle. The SOP (Standard Operating Procedure) dictated that on all hoist missions we would have helicopter gunship support. Well, that SOP went out the window when it came down to saving a life or waiting 30 minutes for the gunships to show up. You can guess what we did... ignored the SOP.

This is a good place as any to discuss briefly the enemy we faced. There wasn't just one, it was basically two enemy factions. Both were focused on taking over South Vietnam and return it to a Communist country. The North Vietnamese Army (NVA) were coming from North Vietnam and infiltrating South Vietnam. These would typically be in military uniforms. These individuals were military trained as conventional soldiers. The other enemy faction was the People's Liberation Armed Forces of South Vietnam. These were more like local militia, wearing civilian clothes. I would label this group as Viet Cong (VC or "Charlie" for short). It was virtually impossible to tell them from a regular civilian. They could easily be tending their rice crop with a hoe and then reach down for an AK-47 assault rifle and shoot you. Both groups were armed with Soviet and Chinese weapons of various types, AK-47, to .51 caliber, rocket propelled grenades (RPG) and other weapons. In my experience, I don't think I was ever engaged by the NVA. They were more prevalent north of the area of operation I flew. This is just my opinion based on my experiences, others may disagree, and that's okay.

TAY NINH

This standby remote site was northwest of Long Binh and very close to the Cambodian border. Our living arrangements were a cot in an open GP (General Purpose) Medium tent. You guessed it, no air conditioning. This area was famous for the Michelin rubber tree plantation and a mountain to the northeast called Nui Ba Den. Reportedly, we "owned" the top and the bottom, but the enemy owned the middle and had a complex tunnel system.

I don't recall flying up at this standby location that much, but I can see on my map I brought back, I marked several locations for missions in that area. Obviously, I flew up in that area of operation (AO).

There is one mission that stands out from my days at Tay Ninh. It was late at night, and an urgent mission was radioed in. We were talking with the mission coordinator, trying to get the map coordinates (this is why we needed the map since GPS wasn't around then.) We got the coordinates, but the person we were talking with on the radio was telling us to hold our location until they could authenticate who was requesting a pick-up of an injured soldier. We did this by using an authentication device, KAL-55B. Our coordinator could never get a valid authentication and the mission was aborted. The coordinates were in Cambodia, and we believe it was the North Vietnamese Army trying to lure us into an ambush.

The first time I was shot down was somewhere between Tay Ninh and Long Binh. I don't remember much about it. I was the Peter Pilot (copilot) and still quite new. We began taking enemy fire as we approached the pick-up zone and damage from the enemy's weapons was significant enough to disable the helicopter, and we had to land it in the field. The AC (I don't remember his name) told me to get out and go to the nose of the helicopter, grab the secure radio, pull it out, and head to another helicopter that was waiting for us. We were flown back to Long Binh. I was really too new (FNG – Fucking New Guy) to fully grasp what was going on. I hadn't grasped the concept that there was someone on the ground trying to kill me. I mean, what did I do to them?

TAN AN

It seems most of my 4-day standbys were out of Tan An. This was a US Navy river boat base along the Mekong River, Southwest of Saigon. It had a short runway for fixed wing aircraft and a refueling area for helicopters. Our living conditions were another large, screened tent with cots and our helicopter about 50 yards away. One huge advantage of being on a Navy base was the food. The Navy eats well for sure. I recalled if we flew missions late at night and would land in the early mornings, the mess chief would be finishing up fresh doughnuts and cinnamon rolls, nice and warm, fresh out of the oven.

Speaking of food, we were finishing up our 4-day standby and were going to be flying back to Long Binh to switch out crews. The mess chief approached us and inquired whether we could transport another mess chief to a different Navy base located upriver. I told him we were not really a taxi service. He offered ½ case of steaks and ½ case of lobster tails. Another good trade and I became a taxi at that moment. We ate well back in Long Binh.

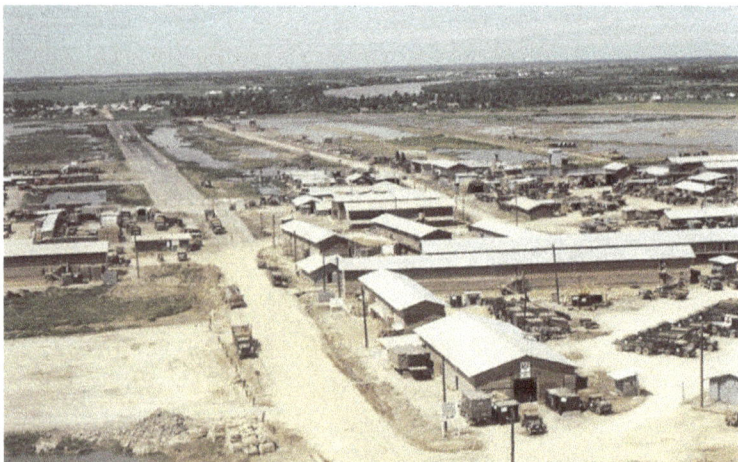

Tan An

Tan An was in the upper part of the Mekong Delta. The terrain was very flat and many rice paddies. Flying 'Nap-Of-The-Earth (NOE), usually 3-5 feet above the ground was typical. Our mission profile was usually this; fly at 1,500 – 2,000 feet AGL (Above Ground Level) to avoid small arms fire while enroute to the pickup zone. Once we arrived in the area of the pick-up, we would radio the ground unit needing us to pick up the injured, to "Pop Smoke." This meant he was to toss a smoke grenade to mark his location. We would look for it and identify the color. We told them not to tell us what color smoke they were going to throw because if the enemy was listening in, they could throw the same color to confuse us and ambush us.

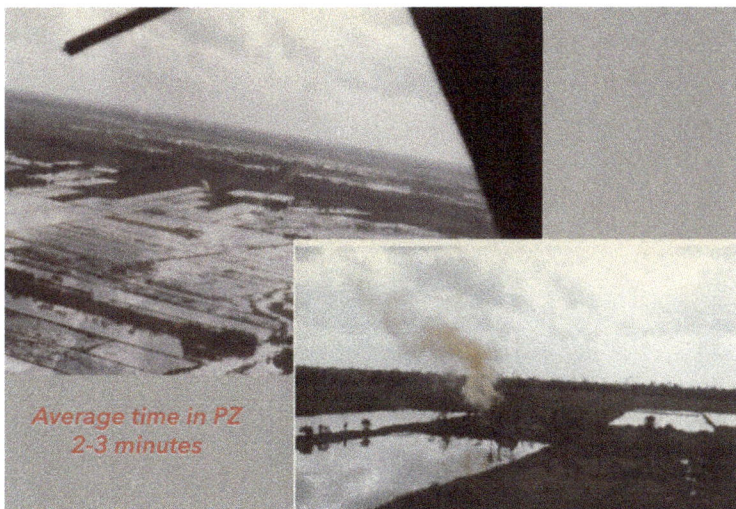

Average time in PZ 2-3 minutes

In the late 60's there was a Kool-Aid commercial that named the flavors; "Cho-Cho Cherry" (red), "Lefty Lemon" (yellow), and "Goofy Grape" (purple). We would use these names to identify the color of the smoke grenade we saw.

(Side Note) I previously mentioned marking mission locations on my laminated map with a grease pencil. I asked one middle school class if they knew what a grease pencil was, and silence. To avoid any confusion, a grease pencil is much like a crayon that was wrapped in a spiral of paper. When we needed to "sharpen" the pencil, to expose more of the black waxy substance, we would just peel away some of the paper away. We would write missions on the windscreen (the windshield of the helicopter); location coordinates, number of injured, urgency of the mission, call sign and radio frequency for the unit on the ground. We would write as many missions as needed on the windscreen and we were finished, we would take a rag and wipe them off. The picture below is Bill Yancey and based on the background of the picture we must have been down south of Saigon. Look carefully at the picture and you can see the missions written in grease pencil on the windscreen.

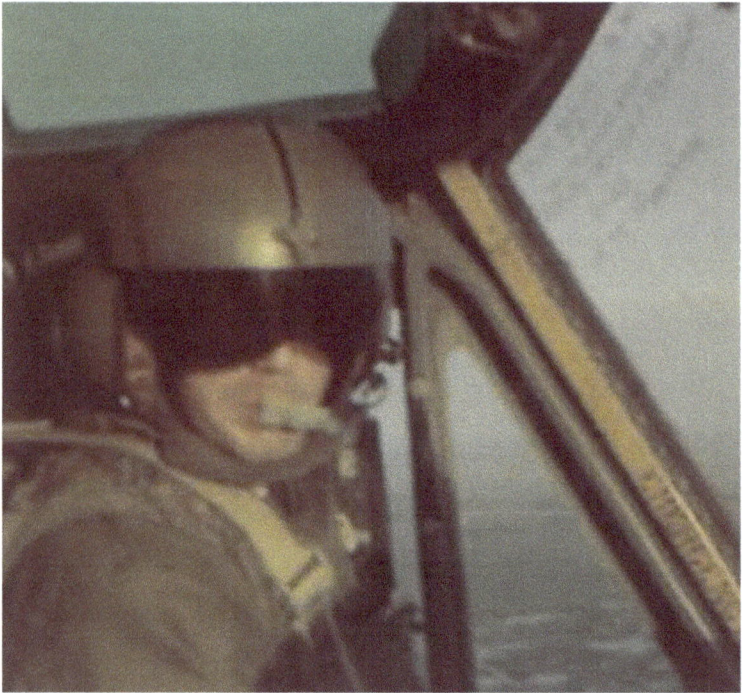

I recall one particular time while at Tan An, the activity was pretty intense, and the missions were constant. We got to the point that we needed another crew to come down from Long Binh to help us with all the missions. This is quite unusual as each standby was typically a single crew, but during this time, we needed a second crew. During a four-day period, one, or both crews were flying missions constantly. We would set one crew down to sleep and get something to eat, while the other crew continued the missions. At the end of the four days, I had flown nearly 50 hours.

MISSION – "X-Ray Sierra 248410"

I was flying with Lt. Jim Ritchie during this standby at Tan An and a night mission was called in for an injured soldier. The location was a small outpost near the Mekong River. We flew toward the location at 1,500 feet until we could locate their location. The outpost was triangular, maybe 100 meters in total width. The ground unit gave us the pertinent information about the patient, enemy contact and the status of the patient. It was a very small pick-up area, and it would be a tight fit. Circling overhead we planned our flight path, and then we began to see red tracers coming up at us. We turned off our external navigation lights. Not really concerned about those since we were still pretty high, but then the crew chief or medic shouted that they could see green tracers now coming up out of the jungle towards us. These were .51 caliber tracers, and much more likely to reach us. Flying in a 'blackout' configuration, they were firing strictly at the sound. We started out of altitude, down to the outpost and landed as quickly as we could, loaded the patient, and expedited our departure. We took a different flight path on the way out and didn't take any more enemy fire. While we took enemy fire going in, I don't recall taking any fire on our way out.

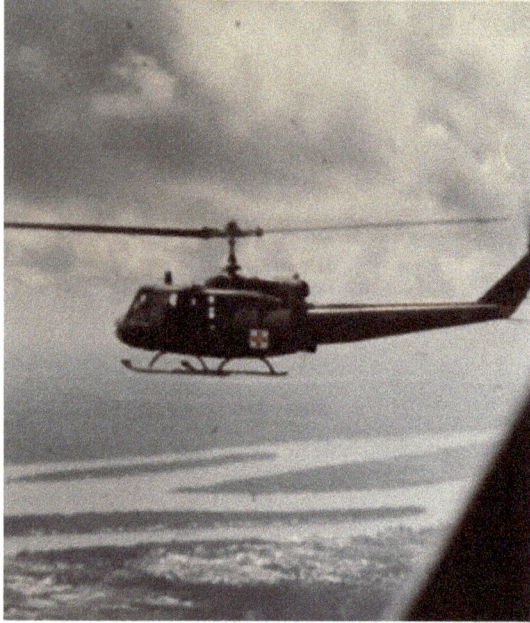

The next day, we got another mission at the same outpost, this time during the daylight. We approached the same pick-up area, and we could clearly see a bunch of antennas and other hazards that we missed the night before. How we didn't hit them the previous night is still a mystery. Has anyone asked yet, if there are so many patients needed to be picked up at this location and enemy contact was minimal, we need to redefine "minimal contact." END OF MISSION

This next story is not part of a mission that I can give much detail to, but it was an event that happened while flying out of Tan An. Before I get into the story, it is important that you should know. First, the Huey could normally fly almost two hours on a full load of fuel. When we would 'hot refuel', meaning that we would land at a refueling station, and not shutdown the engine, just bring it to idle to refuel. While there we could relieve ourselves while standing alongside of the helicopter while the crew chief refueled the aircraft. We would take turns as necessary. The other fact you should know is what a '4x4' is (no it's not lumber, at least not in this story). A '4x4' is a medical first aid gauze pad, that is used for first aid. So now that you know this, here is the story...

It was late at night, probably after midnight and we had just dropped off our patients at My Tho and headed back to Tan An about 30 minutes away. On the intercom my medic said, "Sir? I need to take a shit!" I replied we would be back in about 30 minutes. He said, "I need to take a shit NOW!" I'm thinking, what the hell am I to do? I don't want him pooping in the helicopter... imagine that for a second. So, I said okay. I saw a small village just below us. It had maybe a dozen buildings and just a few lights. Who was there? VC (Viet Cong)? I had no clue, but we had an 'urgent' mission for the medic. There was a narrow dirt road heading east from the village and enough room to land on it. I turned off all my lights and descended to the road.

The medic jumped out as soon as we touched down and went to do his "business." The crew chief was totally freaking out. He grabbed his M-16A just waiting for the VC (Viet Cong) to pop out of one the buildings and start shooting at us. That was a possibility for sure.

The medic was on a 50-foot intercom cord so we could still talk with him. He's out there, in the pitch black on the right side of the helicopter. He calls to the crew chief, "Bring me some more 4x4's!" The crew chief replied with words that are not appropriate to print, but the point was that the medic should come get them himself. "Business" done…we departed a few minutes later, without taking any enemy fire, but left some 4x4's for the locals to dispose of.

MISSION – "X-Ray Sierra 335520"

As I have already mentioned, we flew a lot of missions at night. The technique that I was taught and used was to fly at 1,500 feet AGL to the vicinity of the pickup zone (PZ) with our navigation and rotating beacon on. The ground unit would mark their location with all sorts of devices. During the day, it was easy, a smoke grenade, at night, it was a different story. Sometimes the ground unit would pop a flare, or use a strobe light. It really depended on the enemy situation. The ground unit may not want to bring attention to their location because the proximity of the enemy. At times, the only thing they had was a Zippo lighter, and as dark as it was, it was enough. Once the PZ was identified with a light, we would go black out, turning off all exterior lights, do a crazy maneuver to descend as rapidly as we could, totally blacked out. The reason for our blackout procedure is not to let any enemy forces see us. Once we get close to the ground, I would tell the copilot to turn on the landing light on final approach. Since I flew in the left seat, the copilot controls the landing light switch on his collective. Well, I hadn't called for the light to be turned on yet, as my attention was on something else, but the copilot turned on the landing light. There it was… THE GROUND! The rice paddies, the palm trees, and we were still descending and flying around 80 knots. We were closer to the ground than I thought. I believe God turned on that landing light. We leveled out, flew the remaining short distance to the PZ, landed, turned off the light, loaded our injured, and departed. I would not be writing this story if that landing light had not been turned on when it was. (I almost needed a 4x4 then.) END OF MISSION.

NUI DAT

For any number of reasons, I didn't get too many 4-day standbys at Nui Dat. It was another standby southeast of Saigon. This was a standby site run by the Australians. I don't recall flying very many missions out of Nui Dat, so we had a little more down time than the other sites.

Some of the unique memories of Nui Dat were at 4:00PM, we would have tea. It was time to enjoy a cup of tea, and we were expected to join the Aussies for their tea. Still crazy to think we were sipping tea while in a combat zone. Another memory was that when we went to dinner, there was a white tablecloth on the table, a small menu with two entrée choices, served by staff. Quite different from the cold C-Rations we ate at other locations.

For amusement when not flying, we would find rhinoceros beetles. The male beetle had huge horns on its head, one below the mouth and a larger one on top. These were the size of an extra-large egg. Anyway, we would find a female rhinoceros beetle and put the two in the proximity of each other. They would be screeching loudly until they joined. After consummating their relationship, the male beetle goes off and dies. Poor guy. If he had only known to leave her alone, it could have enjoyed a much longer life.

The Aussies were great to fly for; I just don't have very many memories of missions we did.

XUAN LOC

Xuan Loc was about 40 miles east of Saigon. Our standby location was within the compound of a 105mm artillery fire support base (FSB). Our sleeping arrangements were in a conex container. For those who don't know, a conex container is a small, steel shipping container. There were several that were linked together for our cots, and I believe there was a radio operator close by. In any case, it was not the best living arrangements. I'm thinking there wasn't any air conditioning either.

Gia Ray mountain was just to the east of the compound and was a good reference point as it was the highest point in the area. To the east of it, and all the way to the coast to the South China Sea was nothing, no villages, no lights, just a huge black abyss of heavy thick jungle. Xuan Loc was hoist country. I mention this to set the stage for the missions in the next chapter, Hoist Missions.

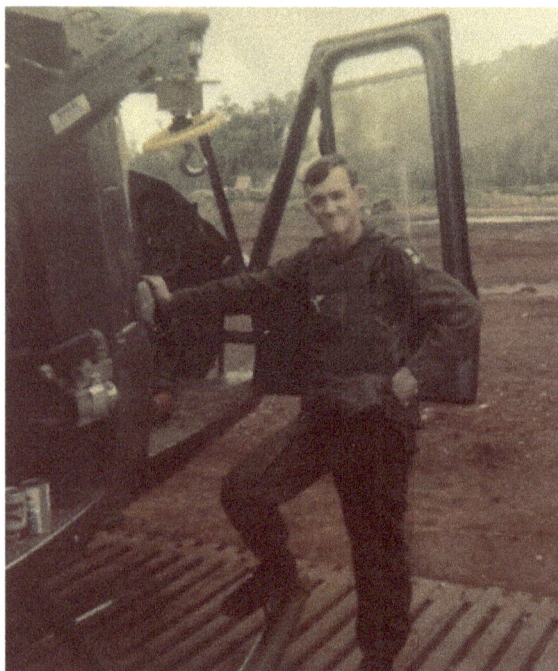

One night the 105mm's were firing for about an hour, I guess. Our conex container was quite close to several of the guns. To hear one of these guns fire, you would hear the boom, followed by the whistling sound of the round, as it streaks toward its target. BOOM… whistle. BOOM… whistle. Whistle… BOOM! WAIT!!! That's backwards. No, it wasn't. The FSB was under attack, and the enemy mortars were coming in. We heard on the radio, "VC in the wire!" which means that the enemy was in the concertina wire surrounding the compound and were trying to get inside the fire support base. This was followed by automatic gun fire. The fire fight was on in a big way. After thirty minutes, maybe an hour, things quieted down and the FSB troops had taken care of the enemy's assault on the compound.

I felt quite helpless. We couldn't rush to the helicopter to fly out of there, that would be stupid. My .38cal revolver wouldn't serve much purpose either, so I trusted the great American soldiers who defended the compound.

HOIST MISSIONS

I made references to hoist missions previously and now is the time to expand on what this is all about. During the Vietnam War there were approximately 8,000 hoist missions conducted throughout the country. It was the most dangerous mission we flew. It was seven times more likely to take enemy fire and be injured or worse. During my tour, I conducted 25 hoist missions, several of which I will go into detail.

At the pick-up location we would be required to hover just above the thick jungle canopy for anywhere from 20 to 30 minutes. We were sitting ducks, easy pickings for any enemy close by. As per the SOP, all hoist missions were to have gunship helicopters to support us. Most of the time, gunships were not readily available, and since time was critical in getting the patient picked up and to a medical facility, I didn't bother to call for gunships. So that SOP was out the window too. Once again, we were out there, all alone by ourselves, sitting ducks, hovering just above the triple-canopy jungle.

A hoist is a mechanical device, mounted on the right-side of the helicopter, just behind the pilot's seat. It can be removed and used in another helicopter, so it's not a permanent device. It has a long steel cable that the crew chief lowered and raised.

We used the hoist when we couldn't land to pick up the injured individuals. Attached to the hook on the hoist we usually had two options, a jungle penetrator or a Stokes litter. We didn't have a wire-basket litter because it takes up too much room in the aircraft. For back injuries, we used the Stokes litter, the disadvantage was the amount of time it took the ground unit to strap the patient into it. Almost every hoist mission I did, I used a jungle penetrator (JP).

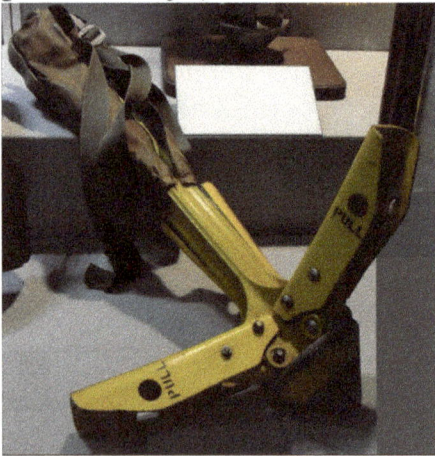

The JP was a yellow painted, torpedo-looking device that would be attached to the hook on the hoist. On it there we three seats that would fold down and a strap to loop around the injured. Even though there were three seats, it was designed for one patient. I had several hoist missions when the ground unit didn't understand that, and attempted to load 2, even 3 patients on the JP. These were usually ARVN's,

(Army of the Republic of Vietnam) but it still caused issues.

Getting into a little discussion of aerodynamics is appropriate at this point. There is something called the center of gravity (CG). It is an imaginary point in which there is complete balance. When a force is applied in one direction, the center of gravity shifts. This is critical to know as it relates to hoist missions. Remember there is a hoist arm extending out the right side of the helicopter and when there is a weight applied to that arm, the CG shifts dramatically. And when the shift occurs, the pilot must compensate with the flight controls to maintain position. The procedure I used was that after the patient was loaded on the JP, I would lift him off the ground first to make sure that I didn't hit the mechanical stop of the cyclic which was keeping us level. After the patient was off the ground, and I still had adequate cyclic control, the crew chief would then continue bringing the patient up to the aircraft with the wench of the hoist. The greater the weight on the hoist and jungle penetrator, the greater shift of CG, and the greater possibility of running out of cyclic control.

MISSION – "Yankee Sierra 290945"

Somewhere east of Saigon, but not as far as Xuan Loc, we got a hoist mission to pick up a scout dog. Scout dogs were a very high priority; in fact, an American soldier was the only priority above a scout dog. Scout dogs were mission critical in many cases.

These animals were being used to sniff out the enemy, boobytraps, and several other critical aspects of the ground unit's mission. My mission was to extract out a scout dog that had been wounded. This was a first for me and we were not exactly sure how this was going to work out. Having an angry, wounded dog running loose in the aircraft was not a pleasant idea. We concluded the dog's handler would sit on the JP and hold the dog as we hoisted them both. Again, not sure how the dog would react to being lifted, the noise of the helicopter, and being wounded was still a concern. As it turned out the dog was muzzled, and we had no incidents after we got them on board and flew them to one of the hospitals with a veterinarian.

(As a side note to this mission, at the 2024 Vietnam Dustoff Association reunion, I overheard one of the crew chiefs talking about hoisting a scout dog on a mission. I had not heard of anyone else doing that type mission, so we concluded Tom Hall was the crew chief on that same mission.) END OF MISSION.

MISSION – "Yankee Sierra 325840"

I don't believe any of us who flew the Dustoff mission became numb to the carnage and brutality of war. Seeing our soldiers wounded so horribly stays with us, even today. When I present my story to groups, I don't focus on what I've seen, just the other details of the mission. This mission is one that I don't share in my presentations. I have tried, and each time I get chocked up, tears well up and I have to stop talking about it.

The mission was in the same vicinity as the scout dog, east of home base, just a different day, a different mission. It was going to be a standard hoist mission, if there was ever a 'standard' hoist mission. As the patient was clearing the top of the jungle, and about 20 feet below the helicopter, we began to take enemy fire. While not that unusual to take enemy fire on a hoist mission, what so hard to erase from my memory was that the enemy was shooting the patient on the hoist as he cleared the jungle. We could see the rounds impacting his body. One after another... He probably took another 5 or 6 gunshots. WHY?! GODDAMMIT! WHY?! YOU MOTHER...!! We got him on board, began treating his injuries, and flew to the hospital as quickly as we could. I don't know if he survived or not. We did our best as what I remember. This image, this mission will be with me until the day I die. War is real... real hard. END OF MISSION.

MISSION – "Yankee Tango 320120"

It was late 1970 and I was 1st up out of Long Binh. A hoist mission came for an American soldier who was wounded. My crew and I sprinted to the helicopter, and we were off, heading east. I forgot to add previously that our missions often took us over active artillery fire bases. It was important that we would not be flying through their firing mission. We would radio each one that was in the vicinity of our flight path to make sure our route was clear. Radio calls made and we were good to go. The concept of "big sky, little bullet" would be a gamble.

Once we got in the vicinity, I contacted the unit on the ground and asked about the patient and any enemy contact. They replied the patient was stable and no enemy contact in the last hour. Still at 1,500 feet AGL, I asked them to pop smoke. We could see red smoke coming up from the jungle. I radioed back to them, "I see Choo-Choo Cherry." They confirmed. Looking at the landmarks around the area, I was evaluating the route in and the route out and briefed the crew. I could see a clearing west of the PZ and made a mental note. We now made a rapid descent from our altitude to the top of the jungle, using terrain references I saw from above, and we began searching for the smoke, all the while talking with the ground unit. Once we approached the top of the jungle, the crew chief and medic would put their intercom on "hot mike" meaning they wouldn't have to press the "talk" button on their microphone (mike) cord to talk. The noise in out helmets was now loud with all the external noise of the helicopter.

I was hovering over the thick green jungle, and I thought I was close to the unit where the red smoke had filtrated up, and the injured soldier, then suddenly, we began taking enemy fire and the rounds were hitting the aircraft. Since the crew was on "hot mike", you could clearly hear the loud crack of an AK-47, in the automatic mode, and the rounds hitting the thin metal of the aircraft. The crew shouted, "WE'RE TAKING FIRE! WE'RE TAKING HITS!" I immediately began a sharp left bank away from the gunfire to get away. I remembered that clearing a couple of kilometers away. The ground unit shouted, "GET OUT OF HERE DUSTOFF 34!"

We had flown directly over the Viet Cong, and he, or they opened up with their AK-47 to bring us down. As I turned the aircraft, I could see our red WARNING lights coming on and it was apparent that we were losing oil to the engine and transmission. The mission now changed; now it was to get my crew to safety before the engine quit, and before we would crash into the jungle. "MAYDAY! MAYDAY! MAYDAY! DUSTOFF 34 GOING DOWN IN THE VICINITY OF YT 320120. MAYDAY! MAYDAY! MAYDAY! DUSTOFF 34 GOING DOWN" was transmitted on GUARD (UHF 243.0), the emergency frequency.

We made it over to the clearing I had seen earlier. We didn't know if it was occupied by the enemy or not. It was my only choice. On edge about where we landed, we were alert to any movement or activity. It was clear that the enemy was in the vicinity, I just didn't know if I had landed in the middle of them. About 15 minutes later, American soldiers in APC (Armored Personnel Carriers) were coming around us and we had other helicopters overhead. We felt a little more secure.

While waiting to be picked up we counted 25 bullet holes in the aircraft, and several in the cockpit where me and the other pilot were sitting. One of the rounds had penetrated the instrument panel and was lodged in one of the instruments, the airspeed indicator, I think. We could see the round in the broken glass of the instrument. If the round had any more velocity, the trajectory would have missed the armored chicken plate of my copilot, and he would have been shot in the head. To say the least, he was pretty shaken up.

About an hour later, we had one of our other crews (probably 2nd Up) land and take us back to Long Binh. Once we landed, I got another helicopter and another crew, and we went back to get the injured soldier. He was still injured and in need to be taken to a medical facility. As I was flying back out, there was a Chinook helicopter with a sling load… the aircraft I left out there hanging below it and was bringing it back to the unit.

Following the same procedure, the same route, but a lightly different approach path to the PZ, we were able to complete the mission, and we got the injured to the hospital. END OF MISSION.

(Side Note) Years later, back in the states, newly married I made a trip to New England for a wedding of one of my wife's cousins. While sitting across the table at the wedding reception, I struck up a conversation with another Vietnam veteran and (long story short at this point), and by our conversation, he was in the unit that I had pulled that guy out of the jungle. He was not the injured soldier but was there on the ground as I lifted his buddy out of there. Small world wouldn't you say?

On November 12, 2016, the day after Veterans Day, I had the honor to do a TEDx talk in San Antonio, Texas. The theme was "Now You Know." About 700 in the audience, were there as I shared this story. Click the QR code to link to that TEDx talk.

MISSION – "Yankee Tango 820090"

As you may recall in the chapter talking about Xuan Loc, I mentioned how dark it was just to the east of that location. Let me repeat, it was DARK! There are no villages of any size, and the jungle was very thick. A mission came in and it was east of Xuan Loc. Flying out of Xuan Loc that night, probably midnight or later, we were flying at our high altitude, talking with the ground unit, we asked him to mark his location. He shot up a parachute flare and we could see where they were. We also had a light ship flying with us. It was another Huey with a Zeon light, that would turn night into day. We asked for another flare, and we turned off our lights, except the rotating beacon so the light ship could see us.

We began to make our descent. We found the ground unit's location, but trying to hover steady enough to do a hoist was a real challenge. Since there isn't any SOP on how to do night hoist missions, we had to come up with our own procedure.

I told the lightship to turn on their light and shine it on top of us. Boy was that a mistake! In the Huey, above each pilot's head is a green plexiglass window. Once the light hit us, the entire cockpit turned green, and we lost all visual reference to the outside. I called out to the lightship, "TURN IT OFF! TURN IT OFF!" Whew! That was close to a disaster. Hovering so close to the jungle was tricky enough, but then to lose all outside visual reference could have been fatal. Gaining our night vision again from that mistake, I called the light ship, and I had him shine the light about 100 meters in front of us, which gave us enough light to steadily hover and to complete the hoist mission. END OF MISSION.

I did another night hoist mission that went a lot smoother. To say the least, night hoist missions in such remote areas tend to give a whole new meaning to "Pucker Factor."

VUNG TAU

The guidance on crew rest was that you were only allowed to fly 100 hours in any given 30-day period.

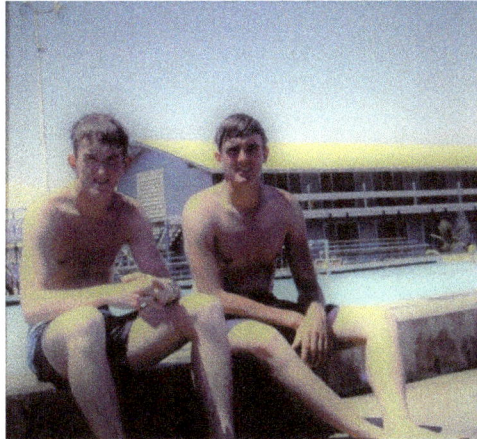

Photo credit Len De Zeeuw

As I mentioned in the Tan An chapter where I flew nearly 50 hours in four days, it was not hard to 'max out' flying hours. So periodically, we would be given time off to relax at a place down in Vung Tau. It was called an in-country R&R (Rest and Relaxation).

There was an Australian recreation site that we could stay. It had a large pool, putt-putt golf course, and the beach was on the South China Sea. Picture above is me (left) with Len De Zeeuw (right), another pilot I flew with.

They even had surfboards we could use if we dared to venture out. There weren't any waves to speak of. 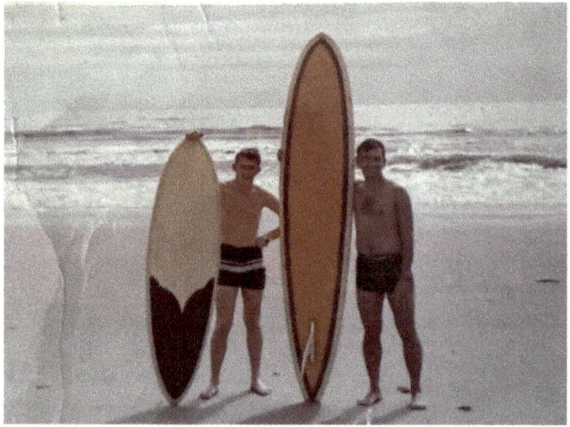 This picture is Ralph Conrad and I waiting for the big waves to roll in.

I think, during my tour, I was able to go down there twice for 2 or 3 days each time.

"ADDITIONAL DUTIES AS REQUIRED"

As with any good job description there is a 'catch-all' labeled, "Additional Duties As Required." Well, being in Vietnam was no exception from having additional things to do other than flying. One of my additional duties was to pick up the movies for the unit from some admin building and show them on the 16mm film projector at our little officer's club we had in the unit area. These were full length motion pictures. Wouldn't you know it, they stopped letting me pick up movies unless I had a U.S. Army projectionist license. Yes, that was a real thing, and I still have it today, though Block Busters never asked for it years later. I was known as "Flick 6" (The term 'Flick' was a term for a movie as most of you already know. The "6" part was the designation of the commander's callsign. So, I was "Flick 6."

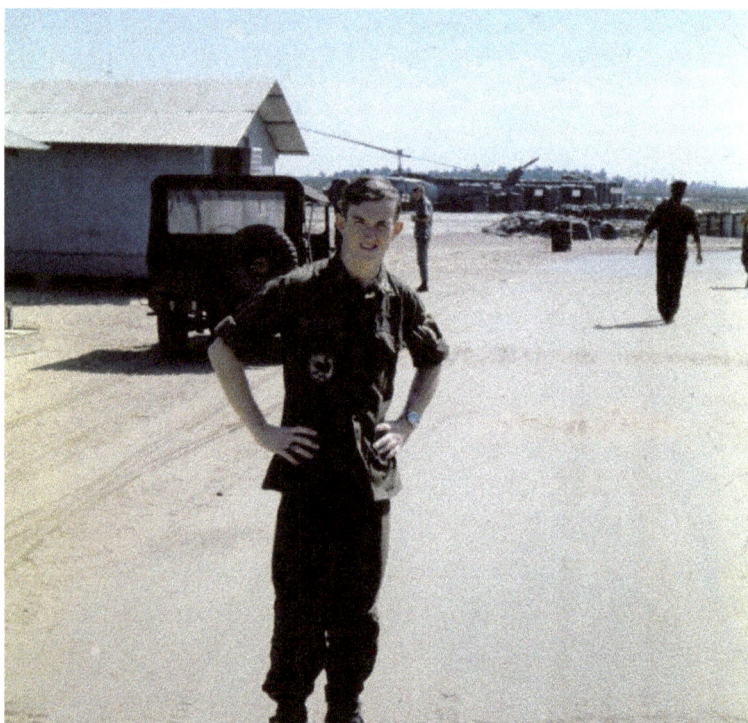

THE PERSON LISTED ON THE OBVERSE SIDE HAS DEMONSTRATED PROFICIENCY
IN THE OPERATION AND CARE OF EQUIPMENT, INDICATED BY (X).

	AS-2 PROJECTOR SET	X	RD-173/UN REPRODUCER
	AS-2 PROJECTOR SET		AN/UIH-2 PUBLIC ADDRESS SET
	AP-4 PROJECTOR		PRINTING & DRY DEVELOPING MACHINE
X	AP-5 PROJECTOR	X	B&H 552EX, 302M
X	AP-9 PROJECTOR	X	AV 900
X	PH 637-( ) PFP OVERHEAD PROJ.	X	NOR CONT 420

AUTHORIZED PROJECTIONIST INSTRUCTOR

WARNING THIS CARD IS NOT TRANSFERABLE	SIGNATURE OF INSTRUCTOR SGT TIMOTHY M. HOEHN

DA FORM 11-78   EDITION OF 1 MAY 1956 WILL BE USED   PROJECTIONIST LICENSE (AR 108-30)

66

Of course, one of the movies that I was able to grab one day was M.A.S.H. and we had a marathon watching it repeatedly until the film sprockets wore out.

Speaking of the little officer's club we had, there was a wall, the length of the building where we had plaques lined up from the "FNG" to "Next." (FNG was already explained, but "Next" was the person who was next to DEROS (Date Expected to Return from Over Seas). The plaques had a helicopter in the center, the person's name, dates of tour, the 45th Med Co insignia, the 44th Med Bde insignia, a banner on top with VIETNAM, USARV patch, and whatever else. Yes, you guessed it, it was now one of my other 'additional duties'. I had to go to Saigon and have these plaques made as new pilots came to the unit. Oh, the fun, driving in a quarter-ton Jeep to Saigon from Long Binh to order and pick them up.

UNIT DEACTIVATION

My DEROS was set for some time in June 1971. The 45th Med Co. was being deactivated in April 1971, and the decision was made that I would <u>not</u> be assigned to the unit coming in to take over our unit's mission. What to do now? I had another five weeks before I was scheduled to return home, so I was turned into a 'gopher' (go for this, go for that.)

One day our First Sergeant came to me and gave me a job to investigate a small vehicle accident in Saigon one of our soldiers was involved in. Apparently, the Vietnamese civilian had filed a claim for damages, and we needed some report, and I was now the designated investigating officer.

Through my thorough investigation, I learned that one of the occupants in the military vehicle was in the hospital in Thailand for some unknown reason. I went to the First Sergeant and told him I needed to go to Thailand to interview this guy. After a few minutes, he gave me the "I see what you're doing Mr. Petersen," look, but still had TDY (temporary duty) orders issued. It was now my job to figure out how to get there.

I was able to hitch a ride on a U-8 (I think) with a one-star general and his aide to Bangkok, Thailand. To cut this story short, I finally interviewed the guy, though I really didn't need to, it was just an excuse to go do something fun with this boring investigation. Now it was time to try to get a ride back to Vietnam. I would check for flights going to Saigon, and Ben Hoa, but nothing. I would call the First Sergeant, "Sorry Top, no flights today." Well, this went on for several days while I had a mini-R&R in Thailand. Then on my morning call, the First Sergeant said, "Mr. Petersen, be here tomorrow, even if you have to walk." "Yes, First Sergeant" was my reply and guess what, there was a flight the next day on a C-47 back to Ben Hoa.

What I didn't know at that time, my DEROS was adjusted, and I was leaving to come home in two days, and I needed to pack and begin my out processing. There was also a going away party that night.

COMING HOME

Like flying over to Vietnam, my memory of flying home is still very vague. I do recall being told that as soon as I got back stateside, it was suggested I get out of my uniform quickly. The Vietnam War was not a popular war and protesting was still happening. Not to bring attention to ourselves (though it wasn't hard to tell who we were), we changed into civilian attire once we were at the stateside airport. I vaguely remember going into the bathroom to change into civilian clothes.

Fast forward to Veterans Day 2018, I was giving one of my presentations to a middle school and, one of the students asked a question, "What was it like when you came home?" To be honest, I wasn't prepared for that question. So many of the earlier questions were quite easy, asking about the helicopter, the weather… whatever. But this one got to me, and I had to take a moment to think of an appropriate response to this very insightful question. I replied, "It's not right for an American to spit on another American." My eyes were beginning to water, and my voice cracked a little. The young student felt bad that she made me cry, and she began to get tears in her eyes too. Once I saw that I told her not to be upset, her question was an excellent question and thanked her for the question. My answer is still true today.

REGRETS, GUILT, AND RESENTMENTS

Some may wonder why I carry some regrets and guilt. More than fifty years later from my time in Vietnam, I regret not flying more missions, not saving more lives. What if I didn't take that in-country R&R in Vung Tau, couldn't I have been taking more missions? What if I extended my tour and been assigned to another DUSTOFF unit and flown more missions. What if...

Guilt... did I do anything wrong that caused someone to lose their life? Did I pull my weight? Did I do all that I could?

Obviously, these questions, and many more, have no answers. I know that, but...

The resentments that I harbor are selfish, and ego-driven. It centers on recognition awards for the missions I flew and the lives I saved. I did not fly any mission with the intent to "winning" a medal. It was my experience though, the medical service corps leadership in Vietnam did not properly recognize the true courage and heroism of the pilots (in particular

73

Warrant Officers), medics, and crew chiefs, who put their lives on the line each time they went into harm's way to save lives. The leadership just felt it was just our "job" and even though we took hostile enemy fire, our crew wounded in some cases, it was just our "job". Bitter, you may ask? HELL Yes! Failure to properly recognize the true courage of these young men, whose average age was 20 was just wrong. Did one of the hundreds of combat missions I flew qualify to be put in for the Distinguished Flying Cross? Bronze Star? Air Medal with "V" device? In my opinion, yes. In the opinion of the "powers to be", I guess not.

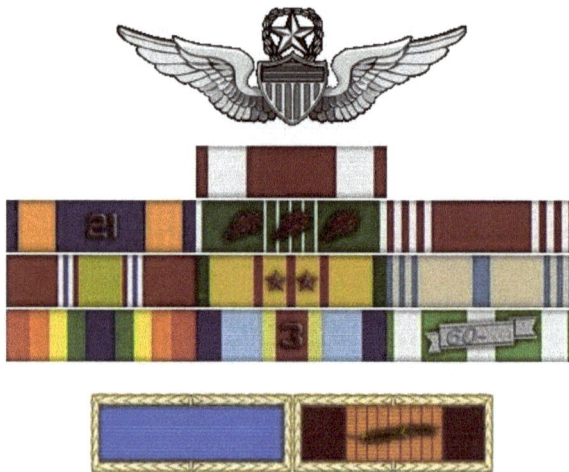

Some of this resentment is tempered with the recent awarding of the Congressional Gold Medal to all the Vietnam War DUSTOFF crew members. The details are in the next chapter.

CONGRESSIONAL GOLD MEDAL PROJECT

Sometime around 2018, US Senator John Cornyn of Texas introduced Senate Bill 2825 (S.2825) in Congress to award all the DUSTOFF crews the Congressional Gold Medal. It was pigeon-holed into committee until 2/3 of the Senate would support it. There weren't any funding issues, and no one could understand what the hold-up was.

The president of the Vietnam Dustoff Association, Steve Vermillion and another individual solicited the support of the law firm Hunton, Andrews, Kurth in Washington, DC. They agreed to provide lobby support, pro bono. So then, Steve asked the association membership to see who would come to Washington and help solicit support from Congress, and I volunteered.

We were a small group, maybe 12 on the first trip and probably close to the same on the second and third trips. The Hunton group had a schedule and list for each of us to visit. We had a lawyer from the law firm as a guide, and we walked the halls of Congress, going into offices, talking with Congressional staffers and sometimes the Representative or Senator, asking to support the bills. There were two bills, one in the House of Representatives, (H.R. 1015) sponsored by Representative Kilmer of Washington and Senator Cornyn's bill in the Senate.

We made three trips to Washington D.C.: November 2023, March 2024, and June 2024, totally at our own expense. With each trip we got a little more support. In May 2024, the Senate passed its version of the bill and in August, the House of Representatives passed their version and was now cleared to go to the President for signature. On September 24, 2024, President Joe Biden signed into law the Dustoff Crews of the Vietnam War Congressional Gold Medal Act, Public Law 118-87.

The Congressional Gold Medal is the highest civilian award that Congress can bestow on an individual or group. It was a tremendous honor to be part of this initiative in recognizing the heroism of all the crews who flew this mission.

In November 2024, the local Dallas/Fort Worth Texas CBS affiliate, CBS 11, news anchor, Doug Dunbar heard of the award and came to my home to do an interview to air on Veterans Day. Here is the

QR Code to the news piece that was aired on the Dallas/Fort Worth station.

The actual gold medal is still in the design phase (as of July 2025) and the actual ceremony may not take place until late 2026, or early 2027. The wheel of bureaucracy is slow and many who would be recipients may no longer be with us.

FINAL APPROACH

We're on final approach and I hope that this writing has given you some insight into my experiences during the Vietnam War. I have left out some insignificant events that really don't add any value to my story. Fifty years later, memories fade, details are not as clear, and I'm sure that my memory of some of the events shared may have impacted the details as I recounted. To the best of my knowledge, what I portrayed in my story is as accurate as I could make it.

To my fellow pilots, our crew chiefs, and our medics, thank you. It was an honor to serve alongside of each of you. If I tried to name all of you, I'm certain I would miss a name or two, so as not to slight any of you, I would just leave it at that.

My final thought is this, I hope by my actions in Vietnam as a Dustoff pilot, taking the injured from the jungles of Vietnam to a medical treatment facility, there is a Vietnam veteran who will sit down to the Thanksgiving dinner table this year with his wife, children, and grandchildren.

APPENDIX/REFERENCES

Public Law 118-87
118th Congress

DUSTOFF CREWS OF THE VIETNAM WAR
CONGRESSIONAL GOLD MEDAL ACT

An Act

To award a Congressional Gold Medal to the United States Army Dustoff crews of the Vietnam War, collectively, in recognition of their extraordinary heroism and life-saving actions in Vietnam.

Be it enacted by the Senate and House of Representatives of the United States of America in Congress assembled.

SECTION 1. SHORT TITLE.

This Act may be cited as the ``Dustoff Crews of the Vietnam War Congressional Gold Medal Act''.

SEC. 2. FINDINGS.

The Congress finds that--

(1) a United States Army Dustoff crewman, including a pilot, crew chief, and medic, is a helicopter crew member who served honorably during the Vietnam War aboard helicopter air ambulances, which were both nondivision and division assets under the radio call signs ``Dustoff'' and ``Medevac'';

(2) Dustoff crews performed aeromedical evacuation for United States, Vietnamese, and allied forces in Southeast Asia from May 1962 through March 1973;

(3) nearing the end of World War II, the United States Army began using helicopters for medical evacuation and years later, during the Korean War, these helicopter air ambulances were responsible for transporting 17,700 United States casualties;

(4) during the Vietnam War, with the use of helicopter air ambulances, United States Army Dustoff crews pioneered the concept of dedicated and rapid medical evacuation and transported almost 900,000 United States, South Vietnamese, and

other allied sick and wounded, as well as wounded enemy forces;

(5) helicopters proved to be a revolutionary tool to assist those injured on the battlefield;

(6) highly skilled and intrepid, Dustoff crews were able to operate the helicopters and land them on almost any terrain in nearly any weather to pick up wounded, after which the Dustoff crews could provide care to these patients while transporting them to ready medical facilities;

(7) the vital work of the Dustoff crews required consistent combat exposure and often proved to be the difference between life and death for wounded personnel;

(8) the revolutionary concept of a dedicated combat life-saving system was cultivated and refined by United States Army Dustoff crews during 11 years of intense conflict in and above the jungles of Southeast Asia;

(9) innovative and resourceful Dustoff crews in Vietnam were responsible for taking the new concept of helicopter medical evacuation, born just a few years earlier, and revolutionizing it to meet and surpass the previously unattainable goal of delivering a battlefield casualty to an operating table within the vaunted ``golden hour'';

(10) some Dustoff units in Vietnam operated so efficiently that they were able to deliver a patient to a waiting medical facility on an average of 50 minutes from the receipt of the mission, which saved the lives of countless personnel in Vietnam, and this legacy continues for modern-day Dustoff crews;

(11) the inherent danger of being a member of a Dustoff crew in Vietnam meant that there was a 1 in 3 chance of being wounded or killed;

(12) many battles during the Vietnam War raged at night, and members of the Dustoff crews often found themselves searching for a landing zone in complete darkness, in bad weather, over mountainous terrain, and all while being the target of intense enemy fire as they attempted to rescue the wounded, which caused Dustoff crews to suffer a rate of aircraft loss that was more than 3 times that of all other types of combat helicopter missions in Vietnam;

(13) the 54th Medical Detachment typified the constant heroism displayed by Dustoff crews in Vietnam, over the span of a 10-month tour, with only 3 flyable helicopters and 40 soldiers in the unit, evacuating 21,435 patients in 8,644 missions while being airborne for 4,832 hours;

(14) collectively, the members of the 54th Medical Detachment earned 78 awards for valor, including 1 Medal of Honor, 1 Distinguished Service Cross, 14 Silver Star Medals, 26 Distinguished Flying Crosses, 2 Bronze Star Medals for valor, 4 Air Medals for valor, 4 Soldier's Medals, and 26 Purple Heart Medals;

(15) the 54th Medical Detachment displayed heroism on a daily basis and set the standard for all Dustoff crews in Vietnam;

(16) 6 members of the 54th Medical Detachment are in the Dustoff Hall of Fame, 3 are in the Army Aviation Hall of Fame, and 1 is the only United States Army aviator in the National Aviation Hall of Fame;

(17) Dustoff crew members are among the most highly decorated soldiers in United States military history;

(18) in early 1964, Major Charles L. Kelly was the Commanding Officer of the 57th Medical Detachment (Helicopter Ambulance), Provisional, in Soc Trang, South Vietnam;

(19) Major Kelly helped to forge the Dustoff call sign into history as one of the most welcomed phrases to be heard over the radio by wounded soldiers in perilous and dire situations;

(20) in 1964, Major Kelly was killed in action as he gallantly maneuvered his aircraft to save a wounded United States soldier and several Vietnamese soldiers and boldly replied, after being warned to stay away from the landing zone due to the ferocity of enemy fire, ``When I have your wounded.'';

(21) General William Westmoreland, Commander of the Military Assistance Command, Vietnam from 1964 to 1968, singled out Major Kelly as an example of ``the greatness of the human spirit'' and highlighted his famous reply as an inspiration to all in combat;

(22) General Creighton Abrams, successor to General Westmoreland from 1968 to 1972, and former Chief of Staff of the United States Army, highlighted the heroism of Dustoff crews, ``A special word about the Dustoffs . . . . Courage above and beyond the call of duty was sort of routine to them. It was a daily thing, part of the way they lived. That's the great part, and it meant so much to every last man who served there. Whether he ever got hurt or not, he knew Dustoff was there.'';

(23) Dustoff crews possessed unique skills and traits that made them highly successful in aeromedical evacuation in Vietnam, including indomitable courage, extraordinary aviation

skill and sound judgment under fire, high-level medical expertise, and an unequaled dedication to the preservation of human life;

(24) members of the United States Armed Forces on the ground in Vietnam had their confidence and battlefield prowess reinforced knowing that there were heroic Dustoff crews just a few minutes from the fight, which was instrumental to their well-being, willingness to fight, and morale;

(25) military families in the United States knew that their loved ones would receive the quickest and best possible care in the event of a war-time injury, thanks to the Dustoff crews;

(26) the willingness of Dustoff crews to also risk their lives to save helpless civilians left an immeasurably positive impression on the people of Vietnam and exemplified the finest United States ideals of compassion and humanity; and

(27) Dustoff crews from the Vietnam War hailed from every State in the United States and represented numerous ethnic, religious, and cultural backgrounds.

SEC. 3. CONGRESSIONAL GOLD MEDAL.

(a) Presentation Authorized.--The Speaker of the House of Representatives and the President pro tempore of the Senate shall make appropriate arrangements for the presentation, on behalf of Congress, of a single gold medal of appropriate design in honor of the Dustoff crews of the Vietnam War, collectively, in recognition of their heroic military service, which saved countless lives and contributed directly to the defense of the United States.

(b) Design and Striking.--For purposes of
the presentation referred to in subsection
(a), the Secretary of the Treasury (referred
to in this Act as the ``Secretary'') shall
strike a gold medal with suitable emblems,
devices, and inscriptions, to be determined by
the Secretary, in consultation with the
Secretary of Defense.

(c) U.S. Army Medical Department Museum.--

(1) In general.--Following the award of
the gold medal in honor of the Dustoff Crews
of the Vietnam War, the gold medal shall be
given to the U.S. Army Medical Department
Museum, where it will be available for display
as appropriate and available for research.

(2) Sense of congress.--It is the sense
of Congress that the U.S. Army Medical
Department Museum should make the gold medal
awarded pursuant to this Act available for
display elsewhere, particularly at appropriate
locations associated with the Vietnam War, and
that preference should be given to locations
affiliated with the U.S. Army Medical
Department Museum.

SEC. 4. DUPLICATE MEDALS.

The Secretary may strike and sell
duplicates in bronze of the gold medal struck
under section 3, at a price sufficient to
cover the costs thereof, including labor,
materials, dies, use of machinery, and
overhead expenses.

SEC. 5. STATUS OF MEDALS.

(a) National Medal.--Medals struck
pursuant to this Act are national medals for

purposes of chapter 51 of title 31, United States Code.

(b) Numismatic Items.--For purposes of sections 5134 and 5136 of title 31, United States Code, all medals struck under this Act shall be considered to be numismatic items.

SEC. 6. AUTHORITY TO USE FUND AMOUNTS; PROCEEDS OF SALE.

(a) Authority To Use Fund Amounts.--There is authorized to be charged against the United States Mint Public Enterprise Fund such amounts as may be necessary to pay for the costs of the medals struck under this Act.

(b) Proceeds of Sale.--Amounts received from the sale of duplicate bronze medals authorized under section 4 shall be deposited into the United States Mint Public Enterprise Fund.

Approved September 26, 2024.

LEGISLATIVE HISTORY--S. 2825:

CONGRESSIONAL RECORD, Vol. 170 (2024):

   May 9, considered and passed Senate.

   Sept. 17, considered and passed House.

BIOGRAPHY OF DOUGLAS N PETERSEN

Doug Petersen grew up on the East Coast and began his lifelong commitment to service early, enrolling in a military college before enlisting in the U.S. Army. He became a helicopter pilot and served as a Dustoff pilot in Vietnam, flying under the call sign *Dustoff 34*. As a decorated Vietnam veteran, Doug flew life-saving missions under fire, rescuing hundreds of wounded soldiers and civilians from the battlefield.

He continued his military career for over 20 years, serving as an Army aviator with assignments across the United States, Vietnam and two tours in Germany. Throughout his service, he flew several aircraft, including the UH-1H Huey, OH-58A Kiowa, UH-60A Blackhawk, C-12, and U-21. Doug was awarded the Congressional Gold Medal— Congress's highest civilian honor—alongside numerous other military decorations, including the Meritorious Service Medal, 21 Air Medals, the Army Commendation Medal with three oak leaf clusters, and the Presidential Unit Citation. He retired as a Chief Warrant Officer – 4 (CW4).

Following his military retirement, Doug dedicated 25 years to the financial services industry, where he helped military families build financial security. His commitment to serving others continued through writing, public speaking, and coaching. Doug is the award-winning author of six inspirational books, three of which received Global eBook Awards in the Inspirational/Visionary Non-Fiction category.

His latest work, *Call Sign: DUSTOFF 34 – Hovering Between Life and Death*, offers a powerful and deeply personal account of his experiences flying medevac missions during the Vietnam War. The book captures the harrowing realities of combat rescue and honors the courage of the Dustoff crews who risked everything "so others may live."

Doug has spoken nationally, including a TEDx talk in San Antonio where he recounted one of his Dustoff missions in Vietnam.

Doug and his wife, Ann, remain actively involved in volunteering with non-profits that support military and veteran families.

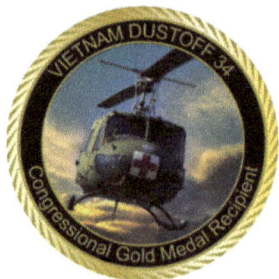

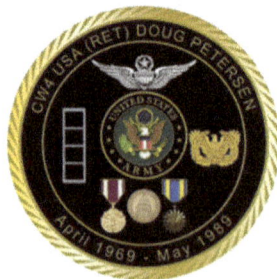

www.ingramcontent.com/pod-product-compliance
Lightning Source LLC
Chambersburg PA
CBHW050823090426
42738CB00020B/3465